CHOOSE YOU

Words to Journey Through
Fear, Courage, Joy, and Gratitude

Mo Jones

For the two greatest gifts who chose me to be their mom—I love you beyond.

Choose You
Words to Journey Through Fear, Courage, Joy, and Gratitude

Author: Mo Jones
Copyright © 2025 by Mo Jones
All Rights Reserved

CONTENTS

JOURNEY ONE
EMBRACING FEAR

JOURNEY TWO
CHOOSING COURAGE

JOURNEY THREE
SEEKING JOY

JOURNEY FOUR
FEELING GRATITUDE

JOURNEY ONE

EMBRACING FEAR

FEAR. How can such a short word with four little letters in it have so much power over us? Just four simple letters with two consonants and two vowels . . . at least it's balanced, right??

This four-letter word can leave us paralyzed. Frozen. We often want to run from fear. Getting as far away as possible. Thinking that the further away fear is, the better off we will be. What we don't realize is, walking toward fear could end up being one of our greatest gifts.

It's been said that fear is often an illusion created in your mind. You create this fear story and allow it to be your guiding light. Guiding you toward the thoughts you have and the decisions you make. Limiting your possibilities. Crippling you in every direction and allowing you to lose your way.

Fear knocks and you welcome it with open arms. Fear speaks and you cower. Fear takes up space and you never question or explore the power of its presence. Why does fear have such a stronghold on us?

It's like FEAR decides to make its presence known, creeps into our minds while we sleep and takes over our bodies. Hi, I am FEAR and I am here to show up for you and do as much damage as I can. Welcome to the fear party. And then, just like that, we join the FEAR party! We join the FEAR party not really knowing how we got invited, and we party along because the party seems like it's so much fun and everyone else is doing it too and so it must be okay. What we don't realize is we don't have to join or attend every party we are invited to! Sometimes, we need to ask ourselves, *is this the kind of party we want in life?*

I wish I could say I have always been able to avoid the fear parties, but I have not. Fear has been a big part of my life and we were showing up at too many parties together.

Let's start with my first day of nursery school. My parents had immigrated their way to the US to live out the American dream. My parents, as many Caribbean parents did, left me and my siblings with my grandmother so they could build their life in the United States. They would work to prepare for me and my siblings to eventually join them.

My first day of nursery school, I remember holding on to my grandmother's hand for dear life and biting my quivering bottom lip at the thought that I would have to leave my grandmother's side for the WHOLE day. All while wondering why she would bring me to this place full of people that I clearly did not know.

Fast forward to sixth grade. I had been living in Brooklyn upon arriving in the United States at six years old. My parents decided to make the move to suburban living and I was going to a new school. Oh, the joys of starting at a new school at eleven years old with students who had been in school together since kindergarten! Talk about fear for my little eleven-year-old self! I had every kind of fear you could imagine.

Fear of fitting in.

Fear of using my voice.

Fear of making friends.

But I was so grateful for oh, sweet Mrs. Ruggiero who could sense my fear so much that she always checked in on me to make sure I was okay.

Soon after, high school made its appearance. You know how they say it's supposed to get better and you're supposed to make high school memories? Well, my high school memories consist of me constantly trying to see where I fit in, judging and doubting myself. Afraid of using my voice (notice the common theme here). Not really having many friends, and a guidance counselor who told me I wasn't college material. Added by a level of fear being my constant shadow.

College came knocking on my door and I thought a whole new adventure would begin. I was going off to college and a whole new me was going to emerge. In fact, the college fear party was so strong I had two chapters of it! And why might you ask?

Fear. Let's start with chapter one. I ended up at a local college. Now, there's nothing wrong with a local college. Local colleges are great for students who want to go to a local college. I, on the other hand, had dreams of going to Johns Hopkins University. I was going to move to Maryland—a state I have always wanted to live in—become a Clinical Psychologist to work with children and live my best Maryland life. Well, what happened?

Fear. Fear happened again.

Fear showed up and robbed me of all those dreams. Staying put at the local college where I was faced with more fear. Two years in, I dealt with a hard time paying for school. Not knowing who to turn to, or how to use my voice and ask for help, I suffered in silence. Attending classes for the last two years, doing ALL the work. And I mean ALL the work. Doing every assignment. Writing every paper. Taking every test. Giving every presentation. But not getting credit for anything.

No credit for my hard work.

No credit for my coursework.

No credit for graduation.

Fear will do a number on you. It will show up to make you think you are not worthy or good enough. The crazy thing with FEAR . . . you can be so riddled by it on a daily basis that you think you are living life.

You get up each day. Do what you are expected to do. And then do it again. Get up. Do. Fear. Repeat. But in reality you are slowly dying inside and losing a part of your soul along the way.

Moving on to chapter two of college life. Remember I said I had two chapters of college life, right?! I was tired of being tired. I knew I had more in me and something was calling me. Was I finally ready to shed some of the fear? I often say you're called to do the work you are meant to do and Speech Language Pathology (shout out to all my SLPs!) was calling me.

Now, I say it's no coincidence that I decided to choose a career that had to do with speaking, expression, and voice. I thought becoming an SLP would allow me to help others find their voice, but in reality, becoming an SLP helped me find *my* voice.

I had to travel my own voice-healing journey. I learned so much about the science of speaking and the power of using my voice. I got to see so many clients who didn't have a voice but who so badly wanted to be able to use theirs. And here I was, holding back! It was definitely a wake-up call that using my voice was a gift. A gift I needed to love, appreciate, nurture, and use over and over again. I realized doing life would require me to fully step into using my voice.

Using my SLP skills and knowledge, I began to explore and tap into my voice. I learned to increase my volume, use more range, and project my voice in ways I had never done. I practiced speaking in the mirror. I practiced using my voice in the car. And I practiced speaking in front of audiences. I took on opportunities that required me to use my voice. Presenting in front of a group. Participating more in meetings. Asking for what I wanted. Embracing fear every step of the way.

But there are two events which further pushed me toward the power of my voice: the birth of my two daughters. Having children has a way of changing you in a way you never thought possible. I now had the immense responsibility of being the role model to show these two little human beings the power of using their voices. And not just for the big chapters of their lives, but also for the simple beauty of the day-to-day experiences that would fill them with joy, happiness, excitement, tears, confusion, doubt and worry. I wanted to be an example for them because when you become a parent, you realize your children watch more than they listen.

I would love to say I had some grandiose event that completely erased fear from my life overnight but I did what most suburban moms of elementary school parents do: I got involved in my kids' school and joined the good ol' PTA! Yes, the Parent Teacher Association.

You're probably thinking, *the PTA*? Let me just say this: don't knock PTAs. Being on the PTA really allows you to use a variety of personal and professional skills. PTA moms (and dads too) know how to get it done. I was pretty proud of my kids' PTA as we did a lot of good work.

The crazy thing is, being on the PTA was something completely out of my element. Yes, I wanted to support my kids' school and be part of making things happen. But I also knew this was a great way for me to really put myself out there in a way I had never done before and work through my own fears.

Remember, I was tired of attending fear parties. I no longer wanted fear to control me. I did not want to spend my days running from fear. I wanted to experience life in different ways without fear dictating what or how I should be.

So, I put myself out there. Taking on roles and opportunities that really required me to show up, embrace fear, and own my authentic voice.

It wasn't always easy because as you know, volunteering can often be a thankless job and everyone in a suburban little community thinks they have better ideas as to how things should be done—but that's for a whole other conversation!

I also found myself finally tapping into other creative parts of me I kept hidden and tucked away. Fear could not keep winning. And I could no longer get caught in the web of what others would think of me. I had creative juices that needed to flow. I started writing. I started a blog. I started a podcast. And I used my Speech Language Pathology expertise and skills to coach women in public speaking. It wasn't always easy. Fear was all over me. But when you listen to the whispers, a flow happens. I put myself out there and what did I discover?

I learned to embrace fear. The fear was going to be there anyway. I might as well learn how to ride with it.

I learned to choose courage. More of that in Journey Two.

I learned to stop playing small. Gosh! How did I dream so small for myself?

I learned to dismantle Perfection Syndrome (more on this later). I am perfectly imperfect just as I am.

I learned I had an audience that wanted to hear from me. People read my words and listened to my podcast!

I kept showing up over and over again. There is no other way to live the truest version of my life.

And I learned to do it my way. All while my children were watching. I knew this journey was not mine alone. Having my daughters watch their mom show up, figure it out, fail, get back up, figure it out some more, succeed and keep going, were the biggest lessons I could teach my girls.

Each time fear showed up, I learned to walk one step at a time out of my comfort zone. I started to become comfortable with being uncomfortable. I answered the call of owning my authentic voice and began to step into the fullness of who I am. Based on my terms and not on a societal prescription of how I was expected to show up.

And each time I showed up, a little layer of fear would peel away, reminding me that while fear was present, it didn't have to take center stage. Fear could AND had to take a back seat. Sometimes fear reminded me I just had to do it afraid. Sometimes I would gently thank fear for showing up and whisper: *I got this*. Other times I danced with fear and we would take some really beautiful steps together.

Now, you don't have to join the PTA, start a podcast, or write a book to embrace fear.

Maybe it's taking a new class.

Maybe it's creating art your way.

Maybe it's using your voice.

Maybe it's starting a business.

Maybe it's learning a new language.

Maybe it's moving to another state or country.

Whatever "IT" is, tap into that.

Tap into fear and let it lead you toward peeling back the layers.

Because embracing fear is not about being perfect or having it all figured out.

It's about being brave, beautiful, and the truest version of . . . YOU.

TIPS TO HELP YOU EMBRACE FEAR AND TURN DOWN THE FEAR PARTY INVITATION:

1. **Acknowledge your fear:** Fear can often be a good thing. It's easy to ignore or run from it, but acknowledging it is the first step to becoming in tune with when or how the fear shows up.
2. **Embrace your fear:** Instead of pushing your fear away, welcome it into your life. Maybe it's time for you to grow and become a better version of yourself. In order to do that, you have to be willing to let go of what no longer serves you. You can't move forward while holding on to past fears that keep you frozen and paralyzed.
3. **Talk to your fear:** Yes, you read that right! Talk to your fear. Thank it for showing up and the lessons you are learning. You can be so quick to wish your fear away that you forget the beautiful lessons that can come with it. Offer up gratitude for fear showing up in your life, pruning and growing you to see the beauty that awaits on the other side.
4. **Journal:** Take time to write down your fears. When you see your fears written down on paper, they might not seem so scary. Describe what the fear looks like and how it makes you feel. What is it keeping you from doing? How does it keep you from showing up in life? Who can you connect with to help you work through your fear? You might find your fear is not as scary once it's written down.
5. **Breathe:** Breathing is the core of our life force. Breathing allows you to calm and regulate your nervous system. When you are about to do something scary, take time to breathe. Breathing will calm your nerves and help bring you back to the present moment to take the next action step.

LET YOUR FEAR BE YOUR SUPERPOWER.

Choose You

IF YOU START TO WORRY ABOUT THINGS YOU CAN'T CONTROL, THEY WILL START TO CONTROL YOU.

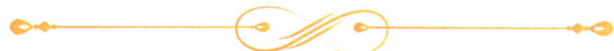

Choose You

GROWTH IS UNCOMFORTABLE.
GROWTH COMES WITH DISCOMFORT.
GET COMFORTABLE WITH BEING UNCOMFORTABLE.
IT IS IN THE DISCOMFORT THE TRUE BEAUTY OF WHO YOU ARE IS REVEALED.

Choose You

FEAR IS THE FRIEND YOU NEVER KNEW YOU NEEDED TO REMIND YOU HOW GREAT YOU CAN BE.

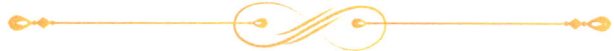

Choose You

THE PAST IS THE PAST.
IT IS DONE.
LET IT GO.
THE FUTURE IS A PLAN.
UNKNOWN.
THE PRESENT IS HERE.
THIS MOMENT.
THE NOW.
BE HERE NOW.

Choose You

PERFECTION IS NOT YOUR REFLECTION IN THE MIRROR.
IT IS AN ILLUSION CREATED BY THE STORY YOU TELL YOURSELF.
IMPERFECTION IS THE HEART OF YOUR SOUL. REVEALING YOUR TRUTH AND LIGHT WITHIN.

Choose You

WHAT WILD, BEAUTIFUL DREAM WOULD YOU CHASE, IF FEAR WAS YOUR FRIEND?

Choose You

YOU WERE NEVER MEANT TO PLAY SMALL.
FIND THE LIGHT WITHIN.
LET IT SHINE. MAKE IT SPARK.

Choose You

I AM BIGGER THAN MY FEARS.

Choose You

EMBRACE FEAR. CHOOSE COURAGE.

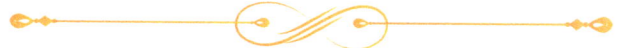

Choose You

JOURNEY TWO

CHOOSING COURAGE

I often say courage is where the magic begins. It is that moment where you begin to embrace fear, step out of your comfort zone, start taking action and doing it afraid every step of the way. Courage is when you begin to finally believe that what awaits you on the other side is worth every step of the unknown journey. It does not promise perfection. It does not promise an easy road. It does promise that you will come out on the other side even better than when you started.

You may think you are born with all the courage you will ever need. In reality, courage is like a muscle. It requires working at it day in, day out to grow those courage muscles so you get more courageous each day and with each experience. It requires you putting yourself in uncomfortable spaces in order to feel that knot within your stomach, your sweaty palms, and hands shaking. Wondering what the heck you are doing while knowing you are about to embark on a soul rising journey.

Courage can often come in the biggest and smallest ways. Big courage often requires a big leap of faith. Jumping all in to take the action to get you from one to one hundred. It's packing your bags and moving across the country to a place where you know no one. It's ending a relationship that no longer serves your heart and soul or quitting that job because you know it's time to go fully into the business that has been calling you. It's writing that book that has been whispering to you for so many years. Big courage is needed for those moments. It's no longer about sitting on the sidelines and watching life go by. You know at your core taking these big courageous steps will have you journey into unknown territories and land you in the most beautiful spaces.

Many times we think courage is only about taking big bold steps. And there are certainly times in life where big courage is needed to grow you to the next level. However, small courage can be just as mighty and powerful. Small courage can be what leads you to big courage. It's taking time to pay attention to your mindset and shifting those negative thoughts when they creep up and lie to you about who you are. It's also about undoing the conditioning of how you were taught to live your life. It's being aware about the narrative you tell yourself of not being enough and learning about the power you have to flip the heck out of that script. It's paying for that class you know you need to help you get your business started, or it can simply be opening up your adventurous palette to try a new cuisine!

The thing about courage is it requires us to go within the deepest parts of ourselves. This is not about surface level stuff here. This is about being willing to do the deep work to discover who you truly are and the amazing things you are capable of making happen in your life. It's not about anyone else but you and your journey.

Courage requires us to show up. It's not the I-am-going-to-peek-my-head-out-from-behind-the-curtain type of showing up. It's putting yourself out there and allowing yourself to be seen. Showing up is never easy, especially if you have to put yourself out there for your business, give that speech, start that podcast, or write that book. All these people and eyes looking at you from every direction and judging you every step of the way. And I can guarantee you that will happen! But if you worry about all those judgy people (who needs them, anyway?!), you will miss out on every part of your awesomeness. Let them look. Let them judge! But show up because there is someone out there whose heart you will touch and who needs what you have to offer. Showing up will be hard but think about how much harder your life will be if you keep hiding behind the curtain.

One of the ways of showing up is by being vulnerable. Now, I know what you're thinking already: *I am not showing up and I am certainly not going to be vulnerable!* I get it. Being vulnerable takes a whole lot of heart and not every person is worthy of witnessing your vulnerability. Being vulnerable is about putting yourself out there to honor those parts that have shaped you into the person you are. The good, the bad, the ugly and everything in between. It's embracing your journey and the fullness of who you are.

Vulnerability is a reminder you are not alone in your story. Think about the mom who decides to share how hard parenting is and that she is riding the hot mess express, or the entrepreneur who shares her journey of starting her business, and how she has failed more times than she can count. What about the friend who decides to move all the way around the world and has to learn a new language and culture while navigating life full of fear? Or the friend who finally decides to write the book despite the many starts and stops, doubt, and impostor syndrome? This is how we create connections. This is how we know we learn from one another. This is how we know we are not alone. And this is how we can honor the tender pieces of our hearts.

So many times while traveling the courage journey it can be so easy to get caught up in perfectionism. I like to call it Perfection Syndrome. Now, let me tell you a little bit about Perfection Syndrome.

Perfection Syndrome is about the little girl born with a blank slate without limits or labels. She is free to grow and see all of the beauty life has to offer. This little girl lives carefree and is not thinking about other people's opinions of her. She is not looking to please the world. She is joyful and free to be herself.

Somewhere along the way this little girl gets the message she must strive for perfection in order to feel worthy and loved. She begins to question her choices, dims her light and shrinks into an unrecognizable version of herself. As this little girl grows up, she is slowly losing herself and her authenticity. She plays small. Sacrifices her feelings, thoughts and desires to a life that appears to be perfect, but she is slowly dying inside. And that my friends, is Perfection Syndrome.

It's time to dismantle Perfection Syndrome. Why? Because you can't do vulnerability and perfectionism together. It just can't happen. You have to let go of the notion of living a perfect life. There is no such thing as perfectionism. Trying to constantly live a perfect life will rob you of living your authentic life. And authenticity is the heart of courage. Being true to yourself is where courage lies. It's that space where you have to go within to collect all your beautiful broken parts and discover the truth of who you are.

And it is in that truth where we accept all of our "stuff". Our brokenness, our flaws, and our mistakes—which I like to call lessons, because they allow for a richer, deeper life experience.

These lessons are all part of the courage journey. It is when we cuddle up to these lessons and welcome them in, we can continue to tap into courage. We can let go of perfectionism and accept our "stuff" that has shown up to teach us some beautiful and truthful lessons.

My courage journey has required me to tap into the fullness of who I am. I have had to let go of so much of my own "stuff" to become the woman I am today and do the work I was called to do.

Courage came calling as I began my journey toward personal growth. I have always been fascinated by the bigger and deeper questions of life. I soaked up that kind of information and loved talking to anyone who would want to partake with me in these conversations. Think back to the Oprah Winfrey Show of the nineties when she would have topics on loving yourself, finding your purpose and exploring the soul. This was well before self-love and self-care were part of mainstream discussions. It was like Oprah was speaking to me and peering into my heart and soul. Finally, someone was speaking my language! I could explore these big questions of life without feeling like I was an outsider peeking from behind the curtains.

While the awakening of my soul has been a long and continuous journey, I have learned to embrace my love of personal growth books, discussions, and podcasts. In order to be willing to explore the soul journey, I had to choose courage. Choosing courage required doing the work of learning, discovering, letting go, forgiving, embracing, and loving all the parts of my journey.

It is not always easy, but growth has to be uncomfortable. You know how it goes: *You have to get comfortable with being uncomfortable.* That is the only way change can happen and changing takes courage. And change is hard.

It takes showing up every day, paying attention to your life and thoughts, taking action, and doing it over and over again. I learned to accept all the parts of me that relished this topic, while also doing the work. And let me tell you, this work is not easy. It is constant and never truly ends. You just continue to rise to the next level and the next chapter to learn new lessons and become the next truest version of yourself.

It is this work that has led me to where I am now and writing this book. I discovered my love of writing by chance, but I really think it was all about divine timing. When my younger daughter was in kindergarten, I received a call from the lunch office letting me know her account was at a negative balance, and I needed to replenish funds for her to keep buying lunch. It was one of those robocall messages. Imagine the Darth Vader voice of *I am your father* but instead it said: *Your daughter's account reflects a negative balance. Please replenish funds so your child can eat.* Now, I added the your-child-can-eat part, but you get the idea.

I kept mulling over the message because I knew while my daughter had money in her account, I was sending her to school with lunch every day. How was it possible her lunch account was at a negative balance? Upon picking her up from school, I decided to ask her about what she was eating for lunch. As I began to ask her questions, a sly smile suddenly came across her face. It was as if her little secret plan had been unlocked. It turns out not only was she eating the lunch I had packed for her, but was also buying school lunch! She proceeded to tell me her hunger was so strong, children as far as France could hear her stomach grumble! She went on to add she has six stomachs, so she needed enough food to fill them all. Clearly, two lunches needed to be ordered every day.

Let me paint a picture for you. She was in kindergarten. Five years old. Elementary school lunch periods are usually about twenty-thirty minutes long. In twenty-thrity minutes she had managed to not only eat her home lunch that I had lovingly prepared every morning, but also managed to get on a line to buy the school lunch and eat that too! Most kindergarteners can barely get through one lunch in thirty minutes! My girl managed to not only get through one lunch, but two lunches! Meal, snack, and drink! There was no stopping her appetite.

After discovering my daughter's lunch plans, I kept picturing her little five-year-old self at the lunch table with a feast of two lunches.

One day as I was walking into her school to volunteer in some capacity, I heard a soft whisper with these words: *Write about it*. I was as if someone was speaking to me. Only, there was no actual physical body next to me. Call it God, Universe, Divine, or whichever higher power speaks to you (for me, it's God), but it was as if God was whispering in my ear. All I heard was a voice and it felt like a whisper wrapped up in love.

I remember looking around me and trying to figure out what was going on, only to hear the whisper say again: *Write about it*. It didn't even make sense to me at the time, but all I kept thinking is *I am not even a writer. What does that mean?* The extent of my writing consisted of papers in college and grad school, as well as reports for work. I knew nothing outside of that realm. But somehow I went home and started typing away. I didn't know exactly what I was doing. I just knew enough to know the whisper was strong enough for me to listen. Something within me knew I had to take this step. As strange as it was, it also felt right.

I sat down in front of my computer and words just began to flow. I don't even know how it happened, but there was something inside of me so strong, it came pouring out without effort. There was flow. A flow I could not describe. It felt like a spiritual moment coming from within, but I was being guided in a way beyond the physical moment.

This is why it takes courage to pay attention to your life. Life is always speaking to you. God is always speaking to you. The Universe is always speaking to you. The question is, are you paying attention?

When something is meant for you, or when you are being guided to your path, you don't have to struggle. It's effortless. There is a synergy happening between you and the work. This is what you are meant to be doing. This is the space you are meant to be in. The answer is right there within you. The question is, are you willing to answer the call?

Unfortunately, so many times you get derailed by internal and sideline voices and opinions causing you to question, doubt, and worry. Your internal voice can be the biggest threat to paying attention. You can be so distracted by life or so caught up in your thoughts, you are blinded by the messages being sent your way. Add to this the sideline voices, and you find yourself in a tailspin of chaos. You look to your left and there is some voice telling you that's not possible. You look to your right and another set of voices is judging your every move. Meanwhile, here you are standing in the middle knowing exactly where you are meant to be, but completely allowing your own thoughts and the sideline voices to collide and drown out the very core of who you are.

And I share this with you because I want you to know you are not alone. I have fallen for this too many times. I have doubted myself more times than I can count and worried about other people's opinions more than I should have. Letting my thoughts take over and constantly worrying about what others think. All along the way, completely ignoring the whispers. From not making plays I needed to make, to following the sideline voices, full of struggle and doubt, rather than stepping into the flow.

But there is always another voice available to you. This voice is different. This voice is not here to break you down. This voice is powerful. This voice is strong. And this voice has heart. This voice is a reminder that what you have deep within is way more powerful than those sideline voices. This voice lets you know what is possible. This voice carries you through. This voice helps you do it afraid. This is the voice of choosing courage.

TIPS TO HELP YOU CHOOSE COURAGE OVER AND OVER AGAIN:

1. **Listen to the whispers:** Whispers are like your intuition and we all have intuition. The whispers are always speaking to you and guiding you to where you need to be. This could be in your personal life, relationships, business or anything in between. Remember, life is always speaking to you. Pay attention to the whispers, hunches, or synchronicities because they are always sending you messages that will require you to tap into courage.

2. **Adjust your mindset:** Your mind is one of the most powerful gifts you have. However, you have been so conditioned to think one way, it can be hard to realize that you can adjust your mindset and approach life in a different way. Adjusting your mindset allows you to start thinking about the comfort zone in a new way. You can begin to be open to possibilities, taking risks and understanding that courage can carry you every step of the way.

3. **Get comfortable with being uncomfortable:** You have probably heard this phrase many times. Being comfortable is safe and easy. Being uncomfortable is unknown and scary. Being comfortable with being uncomfortable is where the magic happens. The more you feel the discomfort and uneasiness of trying new things, whatever that might be, the more you are tapping into courage. You will begin to see yourself doing things you never thought possible. Will it always be easy? No, but one small step each day leads to big changes.

4. **Take action:** It can be so easy to be stuck in fear that you don't do anything. The best thing you can do once you embrace fear is to start building your courage muscle and take action. Take one small

action step each day to move you forward. Over time, those small steps lead to big results.

5. **Let go of perfectionism:** Trying to be perfect keeps you stuck. You become focused on creating perfectionism instead of moving forward. Allow yourself to make mistakes. Allow yourself to be messy. Allow yourself to draw outside the lines. You never know the amazing life you will create.

YOU MIGHT THINK YOU ARE BORN WITH ALL THE COURAGE YOU WILL EVER NEED. COURAGE IS LIKE A MUSCLE YOU HAVE TO WORK AT BUILDING TIME AND TIME AGAIN.

Choose You

CHOOSING COURAGE
IS A JOURNEY.
SOMETIMES IT WILL BE EASY
AND YOU WILL HAVE ALL THE
COURAGE YOU NEED.
OTHER TIMES YOU WILL
WONDER WHY YOU CAN'T
MUSTER UP THE COURAGE
TO GET TO THE OTHER SIDE.
MANY TIMES YOU WILL
SURPRISE YOURSELF IN HOW
COURAGEOUS YOU CAN BE
WHEN FACED WITH FEARS
AND CHALLENGES.

Choose You

THERE ARE MOMENTS YOU WILL BE SO FULL OF FEAR HIDING BEHIND COURAGE. THERE WILL BE DAYS YOU WILL CHOOSE COURAGE AND DO IT AFRAID. BUT THERE WILL BE MOMENTS YOU AND COURAGE WILL DANCE TOGETHER AND BE COMPLETELY IN SYNC.

Choose You

YOU HAVE TO
PUT YOURSELF IN
SPACES TO PRACTICE
COURAGE. YOU HAVE
TO CONSISTENTLY
PRACTICE CHOOSING
COURAGE OVER AND
OVER AGAIN.

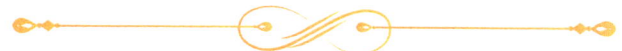

Choose You

IT TAKES COURAGE TO BE ABLE TO STEP INTO YOUR OWN ALIGNMENT. TO BE ABLE TO QUIET THE NOISE THAT SURROUNDS YOU WITH CERTAIN EXPECTATIONS AND IDEALS, SO YOU CAN FULLY ALIGN WITH YOURSELF, IS ONE OF THE MOST COURAGEOUS ACTS YOU CAN TAKE ON.

Choose You

COURAGE IS LOVING
YOURSELF.
ALL OF YOURSELF.
NOT JUST THE GOOD
PARTS, BUT THE MESSY,
JUMBLED, AND NOT
SO PRETTY PARTS TOO.
YEAH, LOVE ALL OF
THAT.

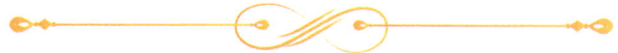

Choose You

COURAGE IS SHOWING UP. TRAVELING THE ADVENTURE. WITH DETOURS AND PIT STOPS ALONG THE WAY. AND COURAGE RISING UP TO MEET YOU IN THE MOST BEAUTIFUL AND UNPREDICTABLE WAY.

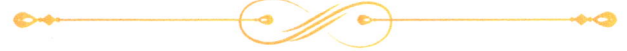

Choose You

THERE ARE CERTAIN TIMES IN YOUR LIFE WHERE BIG COURAGE IS NEEDED TO GROW YOU TO THE NEXT LEVEL.
BUT SMALL COURAGE CAN BE JUST AS MIGHTY AND POWERFUL.

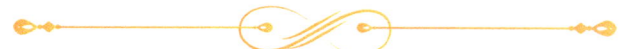

Choose You

WHAT DOES COURAGE MEAN TO YOU?

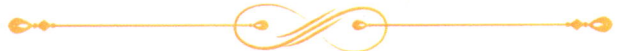

Choose You

MY COURAGE KNOWS NO LIMITS.

Choose You

JOURNEY THREE

SEEKING JOY

Joy. Why is it so hard to let joy in?

Joy is that feeling of sheer pleasure and happiness. That feeling beyond contentment where you are floating in the clouds. That feeling giving you a rush of pure bliss. That feeling that can only be described by three little letters.

Wouldn't we all want some of that?

Somehow joy seems to escape many of us. We want joy. Seek joy. Yet, we never seem to find it or let it in. It's as if we tell ourselves we have to earn joy or work for joy, which could not be further from the truth.

Joy is one of the most beautiful spaces you can be in. Why? Because joy can be found in the simplicities of life. Yes, there is joy in those big life events and milestones. Those are important and should be celebrated. But joy in the most simple moments are reminders that joy is everywhere if we just take the time to pause and take it all in.

So many of us are so busy going through the motions of life, we let joy pass us by. We are so focused on work, school, laundry, cooking, bills, to-do lists, getting here and getting there, we are completely blind to the joy right in front of our eyes. You are not alone. I, too, had been so caught up in the busyness of life, I was letting all this joy pass me by.

For so long, I never even thought about the possibilities of joy. I would go about my day trying to get through being a wife, mom, work, and everything in between. I did not think to look for joy. I did not think I had time for joy. I was so caught up in getting my to-do list checked off, getting through the day, and surviving a life of hustle and bustle, I didn't even see joy as a possibility. Joy was not on my radar.

When you are living a conditioned life and not paying attention to being present, you miss out on a lot of joy. Living a life that tells you to be a good student, go to college, get married, buy the house with the white picket fence, keep working, wait for retirement, and finally retire, you easily fall into a rut and routine of comfort and familiarity. Going through the motions without thinking and without being present.

Here I was married, being a mom, working a full-time job, and I found myself asking if there was more to life. I had gone to college, gotten the degrees, bought the house but felt empty and drained from life. Where was my joy? Why wasn't joy finding its way to me?

For the first time, I began to question if this was the life I wanted. I loved my husband and children, but I just felt there was something more for me. It was really hard to fully figure out exactly what "it" was. I just knew I couldn't' keep living a harried life started by a time-to-make-the-donuts morning (cue the eighties Dunkin Donuts commercial).

I often felt an annoyance toward having to do my morning routine with my kids. I felt it with my job and with life. And my poor husband was often on the receiving end of the annoyance. I could not keep on living like that. Life was supposed to be filled with joy. And I was completely missing out on joy.

The thing with joy is that it really is present all around us. You don't have to buy joy. You don't have to earn joy. Joy is always available. You just have to be present enough to find joy and allow it into your life.

How could I find joy in my days? I knew joy was missing from my life. And I knew I had to do the work to figure out what my next chapter would look like, but in the meantime, couldn't joy find its way into my life?

I began by taking a look at my morning routine. If I could start my day with joy, it would set me up for a more joyful day. I was already working out in the morning but I began to add time for meditation and prayer. This allowed me to get centered and have some quiet moments of time to myself. It allowed me to slow down before facing the busyness of the day. I also discovered enjoying a cup of tea while watching the sunrise was pure joy. I couldn't believe what I had been missing out on. Something as simple as a cup of tea and the sunrise was bringing me joy! Little things we often take for granted.

I also found joy in taking more afternoon walks. After dropping my kids off at their sports activities, I would find time to take walks so I could enjoy the fresh air and be out in nature. Sometimes I would sneak off to a cafe and enjoy a special treat while writing on my laptop. Turns out this is one of my favorite ways I enjoy spending my day. Writing in a cafe. Pure joy. You know what else is pure joy? Watching a smiling baby. Writing in my journal. Dancing to music. Ultimate joy right there.

It's easy to think joy has to be these grandiose acts. But finding joy in the everyday, that's where your heart opens up in ways you never thought possible.

Making time for joy is one of the biggest gifts you can give yourself. Know that you are worthy and deserving of all the joy life has to offer. You get to define your joy. In whatever way that might look like for you. And know that your joy can look different from everyone else.

Just make sure you don't miss out on joy. Let it fill your heart. Let it fill your days. Let it wrap you up like a warm blanket. Let it be your sunshine on a dark and gloomy day. Look for it in the simplest moments. Joy is always there waiting to be found. You just have to look for it so it can rise up to meet you.

Remember, joy is not about having an easy stress-free life. It's about being present. It's about finding those moments throughout the day that bring you peace; especially on the hardest days. Here's to finding new ways to experience the most blissful moments of joy.

TIPS TO HELP YOU FIND MOMENTS OF JOY IN THE DAY-TO-DAY:

1. **Connect with nature:** Go for a walk in the park. Listen to the ocean waves at the beach. Take a hike on a trail and listen to the bird chirping in the trees. Getting out in nature is a great way to find joy. It's a reminder of all the beauty that surrounds you.

2. **Practice mindfulness:** Taking time to meditate, or get quiet allows you to be present. When you are present, you get to feel peaceful, making room for joy to find its way straight to you.

3. **Do something nice for someone:** A small act of kindness is not only joyful for the receiver but it's also a big gift for the giver. When you do something nice for someone, you get to put a smile on a person's face. It fills you up with joy watching someone else filled with joy. Spread the joy!

4. **Find a hobby:** Do something for fun that makes you happy and brings you joy. Whether it's dancing, singing karaoke, gardening, cooking, reading, painting, or writing in a cafe. Whatever that looks like, if it brings you joy, make it part of your daily or weekly routine. Let it fill you up with joy.

5. **Connect with others:** Surround yourself with your people who cheer you on, support you, and make you laugh. When you build these connections they are a lifeforce to your joy. Making memories, laughing, and spending quality time with your people is the heart of joy. And that kind of joy is invaluable. Make time to connect with your people!

YOU ARE WORTHY AND
DESERVING OF
ALL THE JOY LIFE HAS
TO OFFER.

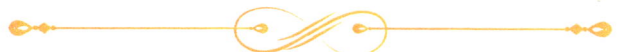

Choose You

THE SMALLEST MOMENT OF JOY OPENS YOUR HEART IN THE BIGGEST WAYS.

Choose You

THERE ARE MILESTONE MOMENTS OF BIG JOY THAT DESERVE TO BE CELEBRATED. BUT DOING LIFE IS ABOUT FINDING JOY IN THE EVERYDAY.

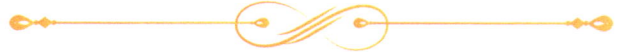

Choose You

FIND YOUR JOY.

Choose You

THE BEAUTY OF JOY IS THE WAY IT TRANSFORMS THE PRESENT MOMENT. THE BEAUTY OF JOY IS IN THE SIMPLEST MOMENTS. THE BEAUTY OF JOY IS THAT BEAUTIFUL MOMENTS ARE AVAILABLE TO EVERYONE. ALL DAY. EVERY DAY. EVERYWHERE. AT ALL TIMES.

Choose You

THE BEAUTY OF JOY IS THAT IT BRINGS PEOPLE TOGETHER.

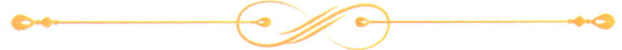

Choose You

BE THE JOY IN SOMEONE'S DAY.

Choose You

JOY. JOY. JOY. OH HAPPY JOY.

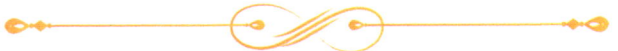

Choose You

JOY FILLS YOUR
DAY WITH PEACE.
JOY FILLS A ROOM
WITH LAUGHTER.
JOY FILLS YOUR HEART
WITH LOVE.

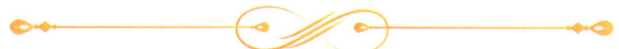

Choose You

JOURNEY FOUR

FEELING GRATITUDE

I have a sign on my kitchen wall that reads: *There is always something to be grateful for.* I have had this sign for more than ten years, but it has really taken on new meaning in the past three to four years.

Gratitude is one of those words we hear so often and apply in our everyday routine. We say thank you when someone holds a door for us. We say thank you after we make a purchase. We say thank you after the waitress serves our food. We remind our kids to say thank you. But do we ever truly take time to truly feel grateful? A deep, heartfelt, you-feel-alive-in-spite-of-what-is-going-on-in-your-life-and-you-are-able-to-maintain-a-state-of-gratitude type of gratefulness? That kind of gratitude.

About three years ago, I started to pay attention to how I was showing up in the gratitude space. Yes, I was grateful for my life, my husband and children, but was I truly feeling and practicing gratitude?

One day I was listening to a motivational speaker and she mentioned how spending your day constantly complaining about what you don't have or what's not working in your life blocks you from experiencing true gratitude and allowing more abundance to come into your life. I suddenly had an aha moment.

Here I was saying thank you throughout my day but finding myself constantly complaining about how I was not happy in my life and my job. Every day I would come home and complain about how work was dragging me down and how much I hated it. I complained about having to get up early in the morning. I complained about dropping the kids off. I complained about how worked sucked the energy out of me. And all that complaining just led to more complaining. Complaining about my house. Complaining about feeling stuck. And complaining about anything that annoyed me. What kind of life was I living? How could I be working on personal growth and living such an ungrateful life?

I knew something had to change. I could not continue to live in complaint city and expect to be happy. Nothing was going to change until I changed. Now, change did not come overnight. My revelation began as I started to pay attention to my thoughts and words. While there were things out of my control, I could focus on the things I could control. I could control my thoughts, my actions, my attitude and my gratitude.

By paying attention, I realized how much complaining was happening in my life. Being aware allowed me to be more conscious and present. As I became more aware, I thought about flipping my thoughts. If I found myself complaining, I would ask myself: *What could I be grateful for in the midst of my complaining?* Even if it was as small as the water I was drinking, or the apple I just ate, or the clothes I was wearing for the day. If I complained about a situation, I would try to look for the good. Remember my sign, *There is always something to be grateful for*? Well, that's when I realized how impactful those words were to showing up with gratitude.

I began keeping a gratitude journal—something I had practiced back in my twenties, but that completely fell to the wayside when *lifing* and raising kids took center stage. Taking time to express daily gratitude for the simplest things and moments in my life allowed me to see how much I truly had to be grateful for. I began to enter into a space of allowing gratitude in. My heart softened and complaining began to take more of a backseat.

Now, this doesn't mean life was perfect and I had zero complaints. I am human after all! But there was a shift in my spirit and perspective to being more present in my life. Knowing that while I was working toward a change in my life and areas I wanted to work on, I could be grateful for what is. Right where I am. At this moment.

By keeping a gratitude journal, I felt more peace and comfort after the long days. And my gratitude journal opened up the pathway for abundance. When you decide to experience gratitude, it's funny how life rises up to meet you. Why? Because when you begin to see life with a different lens, opportunities and possibilities show up in ways you never thought possible. Your days are a little brighter. You don't let things annoy you as much. And your heart is more open to receiving.

I was able to appreciate moments of life in a new way. And I appreciated my life on a different level. Again, not a perfect life. But a life filled with gratitude for the beautiful simplicities. If I was running late to an event, rather than being crazy stressed about it, I would take some deep breaths and think maybe I avoided a potential accident. If I had a tough moment at work, I would remind myself this was temporary and it would pass. If I was overwhelmed with my kids' schedules, I reminded myself these moments wouldn't last for long.

Gratitude. Something so simple but easily overlooked. It is often the foundation for showing up for life. If you can't find anything to be grateful for, how do you do life? Now, there are times when life's moments are so rough and raw, it can be hard to feel gratitude. Losing a loved one. Definitely hard to find gratitude there. Losing a job and not knowing how you are going to feed your family. Hard to find gratitude. Receiving a scary diagnosis. Hard to find gratitude there. And while I don't have all the answers, I do think the smallest seeds of gratitude can help you travel life's most challenging roads.

It's also important to be gentle and kind with yourself as you begin your gratitude journey. Remember, it's a journey for a reason. You don't just wake up with new thoughts, suddenly stop complaining and have all the gratitude in your heart. That's why it's called a practice. It's about working on it every day so that it becomes a part of your daily life. Some days will be better than others. But if you stay the course, you will find how much gratitude is in your heart for all that life has to offer.

TIPS TO HELP YOU PRACTICE GRATITUDE IN YOUR DAY-TO-DAY:

1. **Get quiet:** Take some time to slow down and reflect on what you are thankful for. When you can get still and quiet, you are able to be present in the moment for gratitude to enter your heart space. Let your thoughts fill you up and remind you of the beautiful life you have.
2. **Start a gratitude journal:** Take time to write down what you are grateful for. Start by writing three things you are grateful for and adding to it each day. You'll be surprised how much gratitude you have in your life.
3. **Be specific:** Find specific things you are grateful for in your life. Instead of saying that *I am grateful for my health*, say *I am grateful for my legs that allow me to walk, run and climb the stairs*. When you can get specific, it allows you to dive deeper into gratitude.
4. **Share gratitude with others:** Take time to express gratitude to those in your life. Thank them for their presence in your life and what they mean to you. It will not only be meaningful for them, but it will also fill you up by creating a ripple effect of gratitude.
5. **Be consistent:** Make practicing gratitude a part of your daily routine. Having a consistent gratitude practice really helps you see what's really important. You begin to appreciate the little moments life has to offer. And when life throws you some curveballs, you have a toolkit to help you navigate the journey.

GRATITUDE IS THE SILVER LINING OF A HARD DAY.

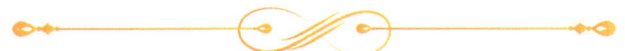

Choose You

GRATITUDE SHIFTS YOUR MINDSET FROM WISHING FOR WHAT COULD BE TO ACCEPTING THE PRESENT FOR WHAT IS.

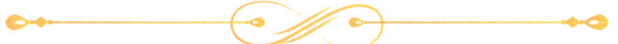

Choose You

THE MORE GRATITUDE YOU HAVE, THE MORE LIFE RISES UP TO MEET YOU.

Choose You

GRATITUDE. THAT'S WHERE IT'S AT.

Choose You

I HOPE YOU CHOOSE GRATITUDE.

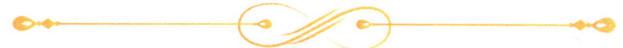

Choose You

PRACTICE GRATITUDE
ON YOUR TOUGH DAYS.
PRACTICE GRATITUDE
ON YOUR EASY DAYS.
JUST DON'T STOP
PRACTICING
GRATITUDE.

Choose You

WHEN YOU PRACTICE GRATITUDE, YOUR EYES AND HEART OPEN UP TO NEW POSSIBILITIES.

Choose You

LET GRATITUDE SERVE YOU WELL.

Choose You

GRATITUDE FEEDS YOUR SOUL AND SOOTHES YOUR SPIRIT.

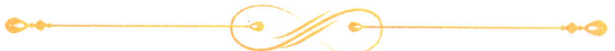

Choose You

GRATITUDE BEGINS WITH YOUR THOUGHTS. IF YOU CAN FLIP YOUR THOUGHTS, GRATITUDE IS RIGHT THERE TO CATCH YOU.

Choose You

THERE IS ALWAYS SOMETHING TO BE GRATEFUL FOR.

Choose You

The Journey Continues . . .

GRATITUDE

Thank you to my husband for your endless love and support. I choose you over and over again.

To my beautiful daughters—you have taught me to give and receive love in a way I never thought possible. Thank you for being my greatest teachers. May you always remember you get to choose you—over and over again.

And to you, the readers—I hope my words inspire your journey. May you always know what's possible for your life when you . . . CHOOSE YOU.

Let's keep doing this together . . . one word at a time.

Mo

ABOUT THE AUTHOR

Mo Jones is a dreamer, writer, podcast host and speaker. Mo didn't wait until everything was perfect to follow her dreams, she said yes in the messy middle. And she's still saying yes. Through her journey, she is choosing courage every step of the way and finding joy is always waiting for her. All while staying rooted in gratitude and dancing through life.

Mo writes to inspire the woman who has a dream tugging at her heart. Her words are a gentle nudge to the power that already lies within you. It's time to stop playing small, start showing up, and live the truest version of your life. It's time to . . . choose you.

To read more of her words,
please visit: www.mojonesspeaks.com.

To join her Friday Dance Parties,
you can follow her on Instagram: @mojonespeaks

www.ingramcontent.com/pod-product-compliance
Lightning Source LLC
Chambersburg PA
CBHW061234070526
44584CB00030B/4125